MS Warrior
Taking Back Your Life After MS

Written By: Danielle Vonn Brandt

About Me

I am Danielle Vonn Brandt. I am an MS Warrior, an EMT, a Fitness Instructor and a lover of all old and funky things. I was born in Port Orchard, Washington but currently live in the Adirondacks on Chateaugay Lake in Upstate New York. I live with my 3 crazy and beautiful children, Hailie, James and Gwyneth, my life partner William, my dog Gunner Blu and my cats Frankie Blu-eyes, Katniss, Cleo and Zuzu. Iwas diagnosed with MS in 2008.

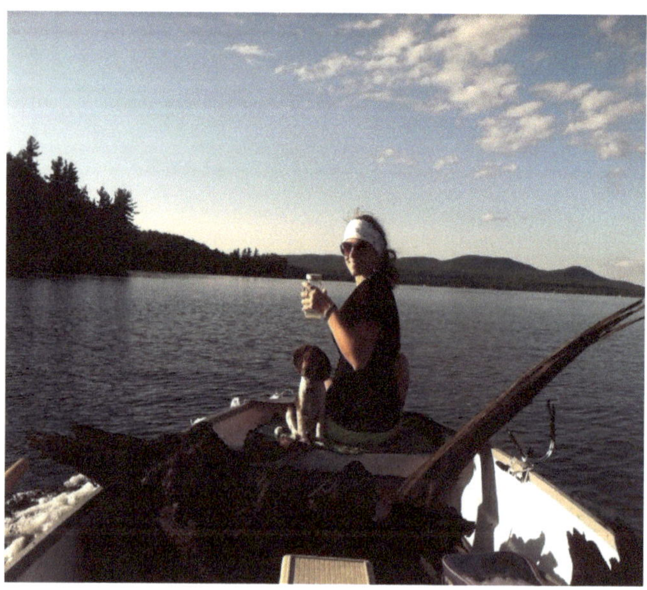

MS Warrior

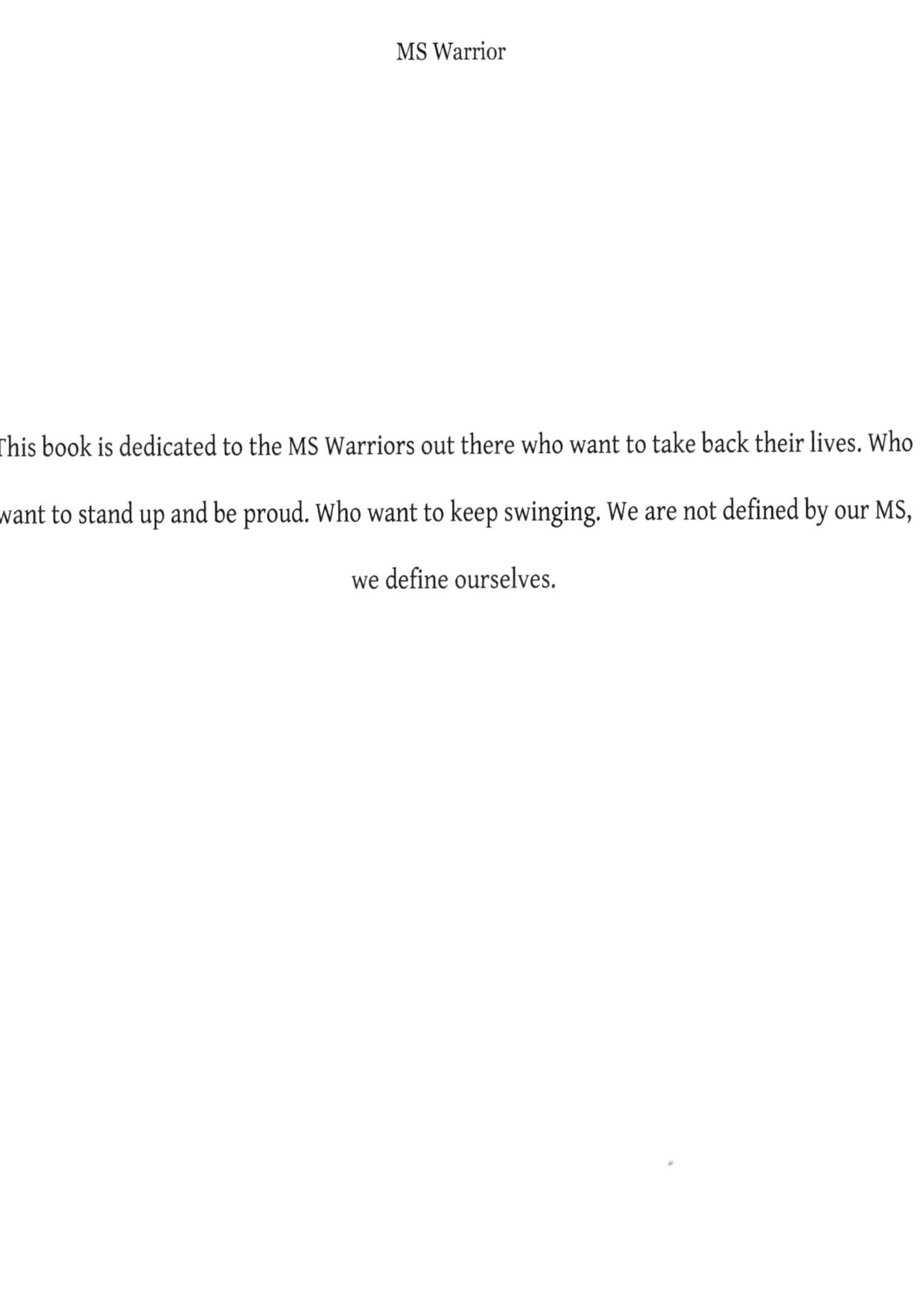

This book is dedicated to the MS Warriors out there who want to take back their lives. Who want to stand up and be proud. Who want to keep swinging. We are not defined by our MS, we define ourselves.

Enough Is Enough

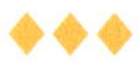

I'm not ashamed of my disease, but I wish I didn't have it.
I haven't done anything to bring it upon myself, but I am doing everything
I can to fight it.
~MMS

OK, so we have MS. So what? We can't change it! We can't cure it yet, I believe that changing our lifestyle habits in regards to how and what we eat, how we adapt and overcome the stresses in our lives (and our state of mind)and always staying as active as we can be, can help us a great deal. I believe that mind, body and food can help us face and recover much quicker or maybe hopefully help prevent any further attacks or at least time in between them.

 We never know when another attack will come, ultimately our goal is to never have another one. MS has already taken so much from us—I think we can all agree on peace of mind at least—why give it anymore? We are not as weak and as hobbled as some of think we are, or other people think we are. Sitting there whining and complaining makes us!

I am there with you and I have been for 10 years, but today is a NEW DAY. Today is the day that we are going to be prepared for whatever it brings. Do you know why? Because we can have control of our lives day by day. Sitting at home feeling scared and sorry for ourselves will not help us (it actually makes us more susceptible to an exacerbation) and no fun to be around. Yes, it is hard. No, it's not fair, but life goes on and we can spend today being a "victim" or start living for tomorrow now.

How are we going to take back control of our lives? We are going to take back what we can control, letting go of what we cannot. We are going to become as healthy as we can be, mentally and physically. We cannot control our MS but we can make ourselves as strong possible so that we can fight back with attitude. *When and if* the day comes where it wants to pop in to say "hello" we will slam the door shut

Our MS is apart of us. It always will be, but I refuse to sit on the sidelines and just wait. It has changed our lives and we can use that as an advantage, since we are already having to accommodate to life with MS, why not just kick start a new version of the life we choose.

The first step to taking back control of our lives is acceptance. We need to accept that we cannot change our circumstances and with that and the understanding that life goes on and we need to go with it. We are **not** afraid of living our lives anymore, we are not afraid of tomorrow. Starting today, we are taking control of what we CAN control!

Who the Heck am I

◆◆◆

I fight like a girl!
~Danielle Vonn Brandt

I am an MS Warrior and my name is Danielle, I am an EMT and a mother. I have been married and divorced. I used to be scared, but not so much anymore. I am my body's advocate, dietitian, personal trainer and mentor. I used to be the "victim" and I was that "complainer" until I realized it did nothing but actually make my MS worse.

I know the words I said earlier were a little harsh, but life can be harsh. Stress, anxiety, constant fear....uhh HELLO!! That is begging for another attack or begging for our MS to transition into a different form. I am not claiming to be an expert on Multiple Sclerosis, but I think we can all agree that anyone with MS has become an expert on their personal bodies. For example, I know when I am not feeling 100% or if I wake up and my body just feels a little off. I can tell I am getting sick before my body exhibits any symptoms because I am that aware of myself. When I am getting stressed or having anxiety, I can feel the numb creeping back—I am comfortable enough to know that I am not having an attack—I just need to step away and calm down. I literally tell myself to stop it, acknowledging to myself that I am in control of my bodies reaction to my mental stresses.

I have had MS for about 10 years and by now I know my personal baselines. I will always push at them, nobody, including myself, will tell me to stop trying to be better. Why are we limiting ourselves. Pushing our boundaries is good for us, not only for state of mind but our confidence in our bodies abilities. Both doctors and ourselves are always trying to fit our MS into a neat little box.. Honestly, most of our boundaries and fears and limitations are self imposed. We need to stop being afraid, we need to shine the light on the shadows *we* have created and we need to push and poke at the boundaries we think we need to live by.

Striving to be a healthier, stronger and happier person will not make our MS worse. Feeding into the fear will. Our bodies feed off of a different drum! Nobody's MS is nice and tidy, it is never going to be the same from one person to the next. MS has its own personality for everyone, which is why we need to stop living inside that box. I know that when I pushed those boundaries and limitations that I had set without realizing it, I smashed them to pieces. It was invigorating and almost magically, that feeling of triumph.

That is what changed my outlook on life as I had currently known! That feeling brought me some much confidence and control back into my life that I decided that I would not live another day living life on the sidelines! That I would not live my life in fear, feeling hopeless and defeated! I decided that when and if my next attack came that I would be as strong and as healthy as I can be. I am not a victim. I don't want people to look at me and see one, and I definitely don't want to be treated like one.

I discovered that when I changed my eating habits and stopped fearing exercise, that I felt my control coming back. I started to pay attention to what I put into my body. Why I needed to change my eating lifestyle and stay away from processed food, sugar injected foods and focus on eating the foods that would help me be healthier. I wanted to understand my bodies relationship with food. The benefits of eating certain foods and watching portion sizes. Our bodies are so temperamental already, why are we feeding it crap. I wanted to understand why I always felt so good after a small workout at home. Why did that workout help to my MS and give me more energy then I have had in a long time? I also wanted to understand how my state of mind and my attitude affected my body, my MS and the way I physically felt. So I spent a lot of time trying to figure it out.

Losing Control

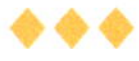

We cannot become what we want by remaining what we are.
~Max Depree

I have lived with multiple sclerosis since 2008. May 17th, 2008 to be exact. It is a day that I will always remember because that is the day that changed my life as I knew it. I had two children at that time, my daughter Hailie was 4 year old and my son James had just turned a years old a few days earlier. Honestly, I was sick longer than my first "obvious" attack. I had been to the doctor several times for my fingers going completely numb off and on. I was fighting extreme fatigue (which I though was due to having a toddler and a newborn) but I was unable to sleep at times. I just didn't feel like myself. I was having constant migraines and my anxiety level was increasing drastically day by day. The doctor I saw several times about these weird symptoms just basically told me that I was "crazy and a hypochondriac" and wrote me prescription for Xanax. She recommended I see a therapist!! Can you believe that?

My then husband had just started a new job and he worked long crazy hours, so I was basically a single mother to two young children. Most of my days just seemed to blend together but that year I remember one day very clearly, my ex-husband had a three day weekend off and was headed to Los Angeles for hockey tournament he was playing in. I remember sitting on the stairs of our condo, crying and begging him to not go. I was such a hot mess, I was terrified about what was happening to me. I knew something was seriously wrong with me but it didn't matter, because apparently to him I was just being a "crazy hypochondriac, remember?

Around that general time frame I drove over to Phoenix to stay with my mother and sister and spend a week there with the kids. It's only a 6 hour drive from San Diego and my grandparents lived in a retirement community in Sun City at the time. We were over at my Grandmas' house visiting with the kids in her beautifully landscaped little backyard.—my grandpa has always had a green thumb not even the Phoenix heat could stop him—drinking her famous sweet sun-tea. I was sitting out on the back porch, in the shade, watching the kids play in a tiny pink plastic swimming pool, it had to be about 116 degrees outside that day. I was sitting there, remarking about how the thumb on my right hand was numb again.

The next morning my routine was the same as any other day, James and I were the first to wake up and so we headed down the stairs to get him changed and get his breakfast ready. At first I felt as though I had slept on my leg wrong, a little numb with some "pins & needles". After I finished changing James diaper on the floor I tried to stand back up and I fell, again I was puzzled but I don't remember mentioning it to my mom and sister. After having a doctor and your husband tell you that you are in denial, you try to keep your mouth shut.

We where headed to the Super Mall that day to visit with other family that had just gotten into AZ. I was pushing the stroller through the mall and my sister remarked about my leg, it was starting to drag. I hadn't really realized that it had been but I did feel the headache brewing behind my eyes. My sister made me go to the hospital, she dropped me off and took the kids back to the apartment.

I literally sat in the ER for about 6 hours before they called me. My mom had gotten off work by that time and came to sit with me. I am currently an EMT and looking back I should have called 911, there have been a couple times in my life that I should have called 911, but oh well. By the time the nurse came out to call me back the feeling and the mobility on my entire right side was just gone, like it had "emptied". I couldn't feel the right side of body, I couldn't stand and my head felt like it was going to explode right off my shoulders. They brought out the *wheelchair,* I had my first genuine experience with a wheelchair. It was not a pleasant experience, nothing like being escorted to your car after leaving the maternity ward.

As you know, there are no definitive tests for Multiple Sclerosis,—in my regards—they had to perform a series of tests and if those tests read a certain way or show some sort of nonsensical probabilities, then you may have MS. Apparently, mine did and I was told that I needed to wait for another attack to happen to finalize my diagnosis. Unfortunately, I was officially diagnosed not long after.

You Are What You Eat

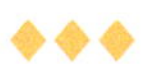

I love food. I do. I love the flavors and the smells. I love all the vibrant colors of the seasonal fruits and vegetables. I love cooking and I honestly enjoy grocery shopping. I love the farmers markets in the summer and fall with all their unique produce that you can't easily find at a grocery store.

But today we live in a society where everything is better fast and easy. They are even turning grocery shopping fast and convenient by allowing customers to literally shop on-line and it is bagged and even dropped off at your home. I understand the infatuation everyone has with convenience foods and fast foods. I have three kids and I used to treat them to Chick-Fil-A or Sonic or Wendy's several times a week because it was easy. I was raising them while my ex-husband worked insane hours and it just made my life that much easier.

But did it really? Yes, it was fast and right there, and it was a double bonus if the place had a playground where they could run their energy out on. But on the other hand looking back, what was I really feeding them? Mechanically processed chicken nuggets and deep fried french fries smothered in salt. Don't forget the BBQ sauce, sweet&sour sauce and the drink which generally was a small soda or some sweet juice because this was a special treat, right?

It has been quite awhile since we have eaten fast food under my watch. First off, it makes my oldest daughters' stomach hurt and she hates it.(Way to go Hailie) Her body is literally telling her not to eat it! Second, there is no nutritional value at all in fast food and it is pumped full of preservatives and has had most of its fiber removed to keep it looking decent, not to mention the fat and cholesterol factors. Companies hype up the savings and the convenience we are getting so that we don't notice that we are putting nothing of nutritional value into our bodies. Our bodies, especially young ones, need actual nutrients. Nutrients we can't find in a happy meal. Third, it can add up financially. Yes, we are paying a lot of money to eat crap that is actually harmful to us.

Super-size my Trans Fats Please

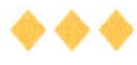

Food we digest can be medicine
or poison, choose wisely!
~Dr. Karen S. Lee

Fast Foods

Fast foods are harmful to our health if eaten on a regular basis and though they are convenient, they are a big contributor to <u>weight gain, inflammation, obesity, diabetes and cardiovascular conditions!</u> Eating fast food can be a very dangerous thing, it affects how we feel on the inside and it affects how we feel on the outside. If it can cause acne and oily skin, imagine the damage being done on the inside of our arteries. The "convenient" Big Mac Meal at McDonald's nutritional information is seriously unreal! Below is a snapshot from the McDonald's website. I was literally blown away. The site also states in tiny print that these are probably not accurate numbers due to all the different locations. Why are we eating anything that will compromise our already compromised bodies?

Processed Foods

Processed foods are another convenience but the act of processing the food removes the nutrients, vitamins and fiber naturally present in the food. It's of no use to our bodies wellness and worst of all, it can actually become extremely harmful. Processed foods are created in laboratories, not nature. The foods are **genetically modified** and may cause <u>gastrointestinal disorders, infertility and can damage our organs</u>. For those who make a regular diet of processed foods, it can make them more prone to being angry and irritable and their bodies are usually screaming for more food not long after you eat it.

Frozen Foods

Frozen meals in the freezer section at your grocery stores are generally high in calories, trans fat (man made fat) salt and sugar content. Again, these foods fit into the processed food category. Just because it is labeled as a healthy and easy option for work or a quick dinner at home after a long day they can can be anything but. **Check the labels!** Companies are very good at hiding unhealthy ingredients by using different lingo.

Wait, What?

Do you know why you are hungry again so quickly? Well, hunger is a message from our brain that we need to fill up on nutrients. Our bodies are running out of fuel, and although we just ate that "super-sized" Big Mac with an extra large fry and an extra large soda, our body did not really receive any of the actual nutrients it needs to keep our body functioning the way it needs to. We are giving our body crap when it is begging for foods that give it energy. Our bodies need energy for everything. In fact our brains use a whooping 20% of our energy. Consumption of natural whole foods can help level out our moods, sustain our energy levels and leave your body feeling full and happy. We aren't hungry again right away because we have satisfied our bodies needs of nutrients. Who knew, right!

Don't dig your grave with your own knife and fork. ~English Proverb

What a lot of people need to realize is that even though we are feeding ourselves everyday, a lot of people are still "starving" their bodies. Our bodies can't survive on foods that have no nutritional value. We are depriving it by not being mindful of what we eat. This compromises our body and our immune system—the part of our body that needs to be as healthy as possible—and will most likely result in other serious health consequences in our futures!

Nutrition Facts

Serving Size 1 Big Mac, 1 large French fries, 1 Large Coke (1,269g)

Amount Per Serving

Calories 1,360	Calories from Fat 520

% Daily Value*

Total Fat 58g	**89%**
Saturated Fat 12g	**58%**
Trans Fat 1.5g	
Cholesterol 80mg	**26%**
Sodium 1,380mg	**57%**
Total Carbohydrate 190g	**63%**
Dietary Fiber 10g	**40%**
Sugars 95g	
Protein 32g	

Vitamin A 8%	•	Vitamin C 20%
Calcium 30%	•	Iron 30%

* Percent Daily Values are based on a 2,000 calorie diet. Your Daily Values may be higher or lower depending on your calorie needs:

		Calories:	2,000	2,500
Total Fat	Less than		65g	80g
Sat Fat	Less than		20g	25g
Cholesterol	Less than		300mg	300mg
Sodium	Less than		2,400mg	2,400mg
Total Carb			300g	375g
Dietary Fiber			25g	30g

Honestly, do we need to add more problems to our list of misfortunes in the health department? We need to look at our eating habits—honestly—and if we find that we are prone to any of these bad eating habits on a regular basis then we need to head in a different direction.

But it's Hard!?!

◆ ◆ ◆

You'll never change your life
until you change something you do daily.
The secret of your success is found in your daily routine.
~unknown

Yes, we live in a hectic world with commitments at work and at home, so how do we find the time to plan, cook and eat healthy when we are so freaking busy? Well, we need to make time. Cut 30 minutes of TV, on your day off, make it a plan to food prep for the whole week. Anything! We have an auto-immune disease. A real and terrible disease where our bodies turn on us. If we want to take back our control we need to put our bodies first! TOUGH LOVE guys, we are going to have MS forever. Do you want to just survive and take it as it comes or do you want to make yourself as healthy and as strong as possible and help your body defend itself.

Our eating habits should be our number one priority. My opinion on figuring out what's healthy and unhealthy is to eat the foods that our ancestors ate. We can pretty much guarantee that they ate fresh ingredients, they are as natural as they come. This generally meant their foods were originally locally grown and raised. I am not pushing for a particular diet like Paleo or Whole30, I'm not calling for a diet at all, just a lifestyle change.

I am just pushing for real food: fruits, vegetables, whole grains, healthy fats, natural sugars, proteins. Fresh ingredients that are available to us. Not canned or boxed or packaged for convenience. I am pretty sure that a hundred years ago they didn't have fast foods restaurants, and convenience stores on every corner.

My 91 year old grandfather told me stories about how he would walk to school everyday with a hot potato in each coat pocket to help keep his hands warm and then he would eat them for his lunch for that day They raised their own livestock for protein and dairy and had gardens for their fruits and vegetables They harvested and/or grew herbs, spices and local berries They didn't have all of these stores stocked full of "easy" foods to grab and go. They ate what was available to them in their area.

We are lucky, today we have it incredibly easy with everything available to us, with the click of a mouse or just simply jumping in the car and driving to the store. Unfortunately there are more unhealthy choices than healthy ones. We have the ability to find whatever our little hearts desire, we just need to know the how and why of foods to make healthier choices. Let focus on fresh produce, fresh meats and whole grains. We'll break it down from there.

Fruits and Vegetables and Grains...oh my!
Complex Carbs and Fiber are a girls best friend.

◆◆◆

Now you are perfectly capable of feeding yourself.
You have plenty of opportunities to
do so, we eat five or six times a day,
everyday of every week of every month of every year.
That adds up to a lot of opportunities to help or harm yourself
~Cameron Diaz, The Body Book

Fresh Fruits

Fruits benefit our bodies immensely as they are a natural sources of vitamins and minerals, which are essential for the proper functioning of the body. They are rich in dietary fiber, which when absorbed with the natural sugars, prevents our blood sugars levels from dramatically spiking. Fruits also helps improve the functioning of our digestive tract and they are an important part of a healthy diet without adding any unnecessary fats. Fruits also help us stay away from health complications like high blood pressure, cancer, heart problems, diabetes and skin disorders. It is always best to eat them raw, fresh and ripe because then you get to experience the real health benefits, rather than consuming them after processing or cooking. They are an amazing snack for a boost of energy and they will feed that sweet tooth (we all have it) when it is begging for something to satisfy it.

Fresh Vegetables

Vegetables are awesome for our digestive track, are low in calories and have no cholesterol. They are rich in antioxidants which keep away diseases like cancer, cardiovascular ailments and strokes. They deliver tons of vitamins, including but definitely not limited to, vitamin A, vitamin K and vitamin B6. Vegetables are actually a preferred source of the nutrients our bodies need vs. supplements. When we are on a diet full of yummy vegetables our internal systems run like a perfect well oiled machine and they help us with our blood pressure, our skeletal system and help us have bowel movements (we all know that can be a side effect of MS). Eating fresh fruits and vegetables will provide you with more of the nutrients needed to give you energy, healthy immune function, and digestive regularity.

Whole Grains

      Whole grains when part of a healthy diet will reduce risk of some chronic diseases. Hmm...I am all about that. They are an important source of nutrients like fiber(again) and our B vitamins and minerals. Dietary fiber from whole grains help reduce blood cholesterol levels and can lower risk the risk of heart disease. What's not to love?

What's important to understand about with whole grains, is that they are still whole! They haven't been refined and stripped of all their nutrients. Lets compare white rice with brown rice or red rice, etc... it is stripped down to basically just its starch, which is not very nutritious. And then they try to fortify it with the same nutrients they went to all that trouble to remove while brown or red rice is still in its natural form with all of its nutrients intake. Same goes for white flour opposed to whole wheat flour. You get the gist. Just because it is labeled refined or fortified that doesn't mean it is healthy. Ask yourself why they had to label it that way?

These three food groups contain our complex carbs. These are good carbs. They make our bodies work harder to break-up them up, which takes time, and in turn gives us longer acting energy and keeps us feeling full for longer!

We will get into the vitamins, minerals, fats and the carbs we need in another chapter. For now, lets keep focusing on our food groups! Next up are our healthy sugars, healthy fats and proteins!

Sugar
The Good and The Bad

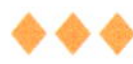

You are so much stronger than you think you are.
~Danielle Vonn Brandt

Let's talk about sugar baby, lets talk about you and me and all the good things and the bad things that can be! Sorry, I was in a singing mood. But anyway, who doesn't love sweet treats? I know I do, but I recommend sticking to natural sugars in regards to our treats. *What does that mean?*

Natural sugars are found in fruits, vegetables, beans, nuts and whole grains and in dairy products, such as milk,cheese and yogurts, these foods provide essential nutrients that keep the body healthy and help prevent disease. Maple syrup and honey are also great natural sources that I use as a substitute when cooking or baking. Yes, you can still treat yourself to homemade baked goods! We want to avoid free sugar as much as possible!

Free Sugar

Free Sugar is sugar that isn't bound to fiber, in like in our fruit and other natural foods, it can lead to inflammation, blood sugar instability and it can, most likely will,over a long period of time, cause type 2 diabetes. If you don't have exercise in your life while your eating all this free sugar, such as sodas,juices, candy and white table sugar, then the likelihood you'll develop these problems goes through the roof. Refined aka "free sugar" causes altered internal pH levels resulting in a more acidic body. It is believed that an acidic environment is a breeding ground for disease, whereas an alkaline body promotes good health. So to correct any type of imbalance, the body draws on its stored minerals, for example, to protect the blood, calcium is drawn from the bones and teeth—enough to weaken our bones —in doing that it precipitates osteoarthritis. Free sugar can even be damaging to our digestive system, particularly for those of us who have difficulty digesting carbohydrates.

I don't buy refined sugars or brown sugars for my kitchen anymore. When I am cooking or baking I substitute **raw honey** or **maple syrup** instead. I actually prefer the taste and love the fact that my food is actually healthier with its natural sugars. There are specific measurements for the substitutions because the it is in a different form and you will not need as much.

EASY *Sugar* CONVERSION CHART

Table Sugar	Raw Honey	Maple Syrup
1 Tablespoon	1 Tablespoon	1 Tablespoon
1/4 Cup	2 Tablespoons	2 Tablespoons
1/2 Cup	1/4 Cup	1/4 Cup
3/4 Cup	3/8 Cup	3/8 Cup
1 Cup	1/2 Cup	1/2 Cup
2 Cups	1 Cup	1 Cup

copyright MSWarrior.org

So, I have recently heard a lot about Agave Nectar, it has been claimed as the new natural alternative to sugar. Well, after doing a ton of research, and compiling a ton of <u>actual facts</u> I have learned some interesting information. This nectar is also known as agave syrup and while it was traditionally used as a natural sugar, the product that ends up on the grocery store shelves is *not a natural product.*

This 100% natural sugar source has been boiled down into thick syrup, much like maple syrup, but it is then processed and refined by treating the natural sugars with heat and enzymes which destroys the beneficial effects of the plant. The end product is a processed syrup, instead of a natural sweetener.

I have reached the conclusion that I will not be trying or using this new *"healthy"* fad sweetener! Remember how I said to be wary about a companies food claims and to read the ingredient and nutritional labels to look for their sneaky verbiage. Take a peek at the chart I made and see exactly why agave nectar is not a healthy substitute and no longer natural at all.

Maple Syrup

per 1 TBSP

Calories	52.2
From Carbs	51.9
Total Carbs	13.4 g
Sugars	11.9 g
Total Fat	-
Omega-6 Fatty Acids	20.0 mg
Calcium	13.4 mg
Magnesium	2.8 mg
Potassium	40.8 mg

Also small levels of:
Zinc, Sodium, Phosphorus,
Iron, Selenium, Manganese

Agave Nectar/Syrup

per 1 TBSP

Calories	80
From Carbs	80
Total Carbs	20.3 g
Sugars	20 g
Total Fat	-
Omega-6 Fatty Acids	-
Calcium	-
Magnesium	-
Potassium	-

NO VITAMINS OR
MINERALS

Stay positive even when you're overwhelmed. Just Keep Breathing!
~Danielle Vonn Brandt

Free sugar

Free sugar is everywhere. It is lurking in all processed foods and can be called all sorts of sneaky names. Watch out for "sugar free" foods, they have omitted free sugars but have replaced them with engineered sweeteners that are (I believe) much worse, like High Fructose Corn Syrup. You want to make sure the labels aren't hiding anything. Even "naturally" flavored juices are loaded with everything but the healthy nutrients from the fruit we are trying to replace.

I know that as a mom I was guilty and naive about the juices I gave my children. Lets not even get into energy drinks and sodas. **Yuck!** Just to point out, I used to be a soda and energy drink fiend—I have since changed my sinful ways and finally realized that I was actually harming my body. In regards, to artificial sweeteners like Sweet&Low, Equal, Splenda, Truvia and Stevia,—well the word artificial should be your first warning— most of these are full of aspartame, saccharin, sucrolose, and acesulfame potassium, which are being used as artificial sweeteners in thousands of products, without us even realizing it.

Actually I was extremely surprised by what I found in my research about artificial sweeteners! Going as far back as 1996, it has been believed that aspartame and other artificial sweeteners where somehow linked to MS and MS symptoms and other brain diseases!

Here is an article written by Russell L. Blaylock, MD, (neurosurgeon) called: **The Connection Between MS And Aspartame;**

Recently, much controversy has surrounded a claim that aspartame may produce an MS-like syndrome. A current review...of scientific studies have disclosed a pathophysiological mechanism to explain this connection. As far back as 1996 it was shown that the lesions produced in the myelin sheath of axons in cases of multiple sclerosis were related to excitatory receptors on the primary cells involved called oligodendroglia. Recent studies have now confirmed what was suspected back then. The loss of myelin sheath on the nerve fibers characteristic of the disease are due to the death of these oligodendroglial cells at the site of the lesions (called plaques). Further, these studies have shown that the death of these important cells is as a result of excessive exposure to excitotoxins at the site of the lesions. Normally, most of these excitotoxins are secreted from microglial immune cells in the central nervous system. This not only destroys these myelin-producing cells it also breaks down the blood-brain barrier (BBB), allowing excitotoxins in the blood stream to enter the site of damage. Aspartame contains the excitotoxin aspartate as 40% of its molecular structure. Numerous studies have shown that consuming aspartame can significantly elevate the excitotoxin level in the blood. There is a common situation during which the excitotoxin exposure is even greater. When aspartate (as aspartame) is combined in the diet with monosodium glutamate (MSG) blood levels are several fold higher than normal. With the BBB damaged... these excitotoxins can freely enter the site of injury,greatly magnifying the damage.
So, we see that dietary excitotoxins, such as aspartame and MSG, can greatly magnify the damage produced in multiple sclerosis. Likewise, excitotoxins have been shown to breakdown the BBB as well.
....we know that about 10% of the population (based on autopsy studies of elderly) have MS lesions without ever developing the full blown disease, a condition called benign MS. A diet high in excitotoxins, such as aspartame, can convert this benign....condition into full-blown clinical MS. The amount of excitotoxins consumed in the average American diet is considerable, as shown by several studies. ...the toxin methanol is also in the aspartame molecule. Methanol is a axon poison. Combined toxicity of the aspartate and the methanol adds up to considerable brain toxicity and can convert benign...MS into full-blown MS. Once the MS becomes full-blown, further consumption of excitotoxins magnifies the toxicity, increasing disability and death."

(Please bear in mind that I am not stating that this is true or that I am a conspiracy theorist! But on top of all the suspicion and controversy that has clouded all these sweeteners since the late 1970's (that have yet to really be debunked) is it really too far off to think that some chemical that is created in a laboratory can be harmful to our bodies? I am just saying that I am skeptical that anything created in a laboratory that has been at odds with safety boards probably isn't good for our body's to ingest on a regular basis. Most other chemicals we ingest usually involve a pharmacy, a prescription and should be taken "as needed" I just believe it should be taken a little more seriously. I highly suggest that you do your own research and come up with your own opinions!)

      I am staggered by the information I found. I honestly had know idea, that what I ate as a child and a young adult may have contributed to my diagnosis of MS. I feel sick to my stomach even as I type this. It isn't like I was an alcoholic, a smoker,or an avid drug user, where at the very least I was making the choice to destroy my body even with all the knowledge we had been given starting as small children in elementary school. I still remember the day that the D.A.R.E team came and showed us kids what smoke from just 1 cigarette did to that fake lung, It scarred me and it was meant to. If I had know about this in my earlier years and avoided these toxins would it have affected me today? Would I still have MS? The power to make that choice was never even afforded to me. These studies and questions have been around for decades but I was never given this knowledge.

      Where is the "scared straight" group that gives nutritional information to children as youngsters. Teaching children what the food groups are not enough. Why? Why? Why, isn't that what kids want to know about everything? They are genuinely interested. They are little sponges and want to know "why"! "Why is it bedtime, mom? Why do I have to eat my green beans... Why does it rain? Why can't I fly like Buzz Lightyear, mom?"

      We would have absorbed good eating habits so much better with a visual and active lesson in why certain foods are bad...not just that they are bad. Why did kids participate in Jump Rope For Heart, aside from it being fun? Where is the knowledge to help prevent future MS patients, or early onset Parkinson's and dementia patients?. What about that knowledge that could potentially prevent you from having the heart attack that causes you to drop dead at 46 because you basically poisoned yourself with unhealthy foods! I mean we teach our children not to talk to strangers, and to use the crosswalk and always look both ways twice before crossing, why they need to buckle-up or wear a helmet! Why is so difficult to teach them why food is so important?

      Why are we not helping our future generations to learn from our mistakes? We need to teach them to have a good healthy relationship with food. We would save ourselves so much time and effort and even grief and loss if we were already living the lifestyle of healthy eating from a young age We can't change the past, but we can learn from it. Knowledge is powerful but it is a personal choice whether we use it or not. I have learned from it, it has changed my life, I am very careful about what I put into my body. Sharing with my children the knowledge I have learned is the best gift I can give them.

Carb, oh, carb
where art thou?

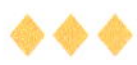

You are one decision away from a totally different life.
~Mark Batterson

Carbs come in two types: complex carbs and simple carbs. They are named aptly and their titles pretty much describe them. The two carbs couldn't be anymore opposite of each other. Carbs get a bad reputation because they aren't fully understood and when we buy breads and other goods, the food labels don't tell us which carbs we will be eating. The key is finding the **right carbs.**

Complex Carbohydrates

Complex carbs are harder for our bodies to break down, which takes time, and in turn gives us longer acting energy and keeps us feeling full for longer! Complex carbs pack in more nutrients than simple carbs, because they are higher in fiber and digest more slowly. They are also ideal for people with diabetes because they help manage post-meal blood sugar spikes.

Good examples of complex carbs are:

- Starchy vegetables like Sweet Potatoes, squashes like Acorn, Butternut, Spaghetti and Pumpkin
- Greens like kale and spinach
- Fruits - fructose
- Milk - lactose
- Quinoa
- Rices unaltered such as brown, red, black, wild
- All Whole Grains
- Garbanzo Beans (chickpeas)
- All Beans like Green, Black, Navy etc.
- Lentils
- All Peas

- Wheat
- Wheat Berries
- Oats and Bran and Millet etc.

Simple Carbohydrates

Simple carbs are sugars and much easier to break down, which will cause a spike in your blood sugar levels. While some of these occur naturally in some foods, most of the simple carbs in the our foods are added after the fact. Mostly processed and fast convenient foods are the culprits Which makes those foods high in caloric intake and not very nutritious. Eating simple carbs in natural foods are perfectly fine in moderation. When baking you can substitute natural sugars, like honey or maple syrup or agave nectar, instead of refined sugars like white or brown sugars and even sugar substitutes that claim to be better for you. When in doubt, stick to natural, not man made.

Fiber

Fiber was mentioned a lot as a nutrient that we get from the fresh fruit, veggies and whole grains we eat. It is a complex carb that our bodies cannot digest, but it's value comes with the exercise it gives our digestive tract and it's help in eliminating wastes from our body so they don't sit in our colon and intestines and become toxic to us. It also has positive affect on cholesterol.

I am going to bare my soul... I have issues with my bowels. Honestly, it's a combination of a birth defect, where my intestines weren't laid correctly (I've since had them relaid) and I have also learned on top of that and my MS, I also literally have an uptight asshole. My sphincter has a hard time relaxing. There I said it! It's out.

True Fact: Did you know that the sphincter is the ONLY muscle in our bodies that relaxes when we "flex it", engage it or bear down?

Starch

Starch is healthy in a balanced diet and starches are a main source of energy. When starchy foods are digested, they are broken down into glucose, which is the main fuel for the body, especially for the brain and the muscles.

Fats: friend or foe?
The Gatekeepers

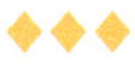

Give me the wisdom to know what must be done
and the courage to do it.
~unknown

Natural Fats: Ironically our body needs them to survive. Fats should account for 20-35% of our daily intake. OK, hold the phone, that doesn't mean go grab something greasy, fatty and fried. We need the essential fatty acids that healthy fats provide us. These fabulous fatty acids help us absorb several—extremely necessary—vitamins A,D,E and K, that's why I call them the Gatekeepers! They are also amazing for our skin, hair and nails, and they give us sustaining fuel for the day and help enhance the flavor and texture of our foods. So lets break-down which fats we should be eating and which we ones we need to stay away from or minimize.

Unsaturated fats: We love unsaturated fats, they remain liquid at room temperature. Our bodies can't make these fats and our bodies have to have them to survive, so we need to include them into our everyday lifestyle. You may be surprised to know that you probably cook with them and ingest them without knowing. They are in nuts and seeds, olive oils, canola and peanut oils, avocados and are found in fish as Omega-3 fatty acids. It has been show that Omega-3 fatty acids are absolutely essential to our brains.

Saturated fats: These are the fats that the world thinks are evil and while a majority of these fats have a bad effect on our bodies, there are a few types of saturated fats that are not bad for us, in moderation, and have some positive effects on our bodies. One that helps with our cholesterol levels is Coconut Oil.

Trans fats: These are literally man-made fats. Although they can naturally occur, it is in very minuscule amounts. Most trans fats we come across today are hydrogenated and man made. Companies created these terrible fats to keep wheir foods on the shelves longer(which means better profits) Margarine and vegetable shortening contain these fats and are in tons of fast foods and processed foods. There is no amount of trans fats that are acceptable.

The most important things to remember when eating fats is to know how much of it you are eating, moderation is key! Making sure that the fats you are eating are the right kinds but not over eating because even good fats can be unhealthy if unbalanced in our diets.

Protein
The building blocks of life

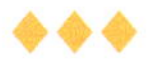

Protein is a part of every cell in your body, honestly there isn't another nutrient that plays as many different roles in our bodies Protein has proven over and over again its importance to us. It is used for the growth and repair of your muscles, bones, skin, tendons, ligaments, hair, eyes and other tissues.

When protein is broken down by our body into its smallest form, you have amino acids. Amino acids are what is used to build and repair every cell in our bodies. Even our DNA even relies on the amino acids found in protein. Our bodies can make several of its own amino acids but there are about eight of them we can't create on our own. They are known as essential amino acids and we must get them from foods we eat. Our bodies require them every single day to stay healthy.

One thing we need to know about amino acids is that our body does not store them like it does when we eat carbs and fats. To make sure we always have amino acids available we should be eating small amounts of protein several times throughout the day. So eating a large serving a protein once a day doesn't really satisfy what our bodies need to keep running smoothly.

Protein isn't just meat

Take a deep breath vegetarians! I got you guys covered! I know that most vegetarians already know this but we may have some new ones among us. There are plenty of other options you can choose from to get the protein you need. Things that are easy to get and from foods that you probably already eat. Foods like Greek yogurt, tofu, lentils, raw almonds, peanut butter, cheese, beans, quinoa, pasta, oats, rices and many many more. Proteins come from animal sources as well as plant sources. Either way, the protein in each source is still broken down into the same amino acids that our bodies need.

One problem I have seen with both vegetarians and carnivores is that they do not get enough protein. You need to train your habits to include enough protein to satisfy your bodies needs. Our bodies need all the nutrients we can give it to keep it on top of its game.

Knowledge is our Weapon
of Mass Protection

"The responsibility to be healthy is in your hands-no one else is going to do it for you.
So ask yourself: do you want to live in a body that allows you to do the things you want to do, a body that is full of health and capability?"

~Cameron Diaz, The Body Book

So now that we have this knowledge in our arsenal, lets apply it. I will go more into depth on whats types of foods fit into our new eating lifestyle. I know that this is a big change. MS is a big disease, and I know the fear that comes with change, with the unknown and with life in general at this point! I want you to know that you are not alone. You have me, your family and friends, and you have a community of other MS Warriors. As warriors, we are all dealing with this disease. It is different for everybody who has it but the lifestyle changes we can make in our lives are all the same. **We can do this. You can do this. Do this for you, for everyone in your life, but mainly for yourself.**

What are nutrients
and why are they good for us?

◆◆◆

Like a wildflower; she spent her days allowing
herself to grow, not many knew of her struggle,
but eventually all knew of her light
~Nikki Rowe

If we want to get literal; here is Websters definition: *a substance that provides nourishment essential for the maintenance of life and for growth*...if you want it broken into easy English then here goes...

Nutrients are **essential** and **mandatory** for being healthy. An essential nutrient is a nutrient that our bodies cannot synthesize on its own, or at least not in adequate amounts. We must provide it in the foods we eat. These nutrients are necessary for the body to function properly.

These essential nutrients include **carbohydrates, proteins, healthy fats, vitamins and minerals (which are found in the fruits and vegetables we eat) and water.** Yes, water is a key ingredient in a happy and healthy life, so chug away. Substituting sodas and sugary drinks do not count as part of our fluids needed.

H2O

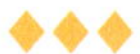

She needed a hero, so that is what she became
~unknown

Lets start with why we need water! Our body uses water in many ways. It cushions and lubricates joints; nourishes and protects the brain, spinal cord and other tissues; it keeps our body temperatures normal; and helps remove waste through perspiration, bowel movements and urination. Humans need to drink water to survive. Our body is approximately 60 percent water, our brain is 70 percent water, and our lungs are nearly 90 percent water. (due to this knowledge I will state that I am a dreamer and like to pretend that we are related to mermaids)

Harsh Truths

When we don't get enough water we will literally die! No really, I am addressing water because it is the most important nutrient of all. It is more important for our body's survival than food. We can only live without water for approximately one week, but we can survive without food for more than a month. Lack of water, or dehydration, reduces the amount of blood in your body, forcing your heart to pump harder in order to deliver oxygen-bearing cells to your muscles. In the early stages of dehydration, you can become dizzy, irritable and have headaches. As dehydration get worse, we will become clumsy and exhausted and our eyesight fades. In the last stages of dehydration, we may feel nauseous and begin vomiting. Without water, you will enter a into a coma and die. Drinking juice, sodas or energy drinks all day are not adequate to keep our body functioning, I promise!

I CHALLENGE YOU! I challenge you to drink 72oz. of actual water everyday for one solid week. I promise you will feel like are in somebody else's body–I'm not kidding–I have already challenged myself and will never be able to not drink a substantial amount of water everyday. The changes it has made for me are undeniable.

But that's a lot of water and I will have pee all the time!

You and I both know you are thinking that right now! **STOP IT.** Yes, you pee, we all pee. It is actually very healthy. Your pee should not be dark or bright yellow, it should be pale yellow. That means that you are getting the right amount of water. You see, your body takes in toxins from everything you eat, drink and even breathe in on a daily basis. Your body needs a way to push these toxins out and replenish itself with fluids.

So basically you drink in water and your body is then able to get rid of whatever stuff it doesn't need or want. Not always is it toxins, even if you are a very healthy eater your body doesn't always need left-over vitamins, so instead of letting them building up in your system, your body simply gets rid of the excess. So drinking water keeps your body toxin free and balanced.

I will make a big pitcher of water with lemons, cucumbers, orange slices, anything I have on hand that I keep in the fridge for added flavor and nutrients. I am a HUGE fan of flavored seltzer water, it has no sugar and no calories because it it just carbonated water. Drinking seltzer made it easy for me to quit soda and other drinks because of that, ice cold fresh "aahhh" after a big slug.

Now that my body is so used to having its water needs met that when I don't have access to water at all times, I find that I get super thirsty! My body honestly demands it! And my goal is to make my body happy. It is the only one I have and the only one I will ever have, so for that, we have become best buddies!

That is our goal, right? I mean why aren't we best friends with our bodies. So our bodies have MS, we can feel sorry for our body or we can help it smash back at MS. All I know for certain is that this is how I want to treat my body. I want to be my body's best friend, to give it the best chance at staying healthy and stronger and happier for longer. I can't think of a better way than that of living my life. A life that I choose.

Vitamin A

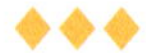

Your only limit is your mind.
~Danielle Vonn Brandt

Vitamin A is most commonly know for promoting good eyesight, also helps support out immune system, it aids in the production of red blood cells and maintaining healthy skin and regulating genetic functions. It also come in variations; **Rentinol, Retinal, Retinioc Acid**

• Retinal: is required for vision

• Rentinol: this form can be "storage" in our bodies and turned in to Retinal when needed

• Retinioc Acid: a growth factor to help regulate our genetic code, It basically can read and translate the language in our genes on what to do and how to do it.

Most fruits carry Vitamin A, but these fruits carry a significant amount and you get more bang for your buck.

Foods rich in Vitamin A

- Carrots
- Iceberg lettuce
- Sweet potatoes
- Cod liver oil
- Red pepper
- Turkey giblets
- Paprika
- Mango
- Whole milk
- Mustard greens
- Butternut squash
- Basil
- Kale
- Cheddar Cheese
- Hard Boiled Eggs
- Cantaloupe
- Turnip Greens
- Pea
- Apricots
- Tomatoes
- Marjoram
- Spinach
- Papaya
- Red Bell Peppers
- Dandelions
- Liver
- Mackerel
- Salmon
- Goat cheese
- Trout
- Grapefruit

Vitamin B

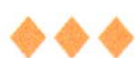

It's OK to be scared. Being scared means you
are about to do something really, really brave.
~unknown

B Vitamins: There are eight B-family vitamins, they include B1, B2, B3, B5, B6, B9, B12. I'll go over each ones. They are also known by other names.

Foods rich in Vitamin B

- Liver
- Peanuts
- Mushrooms
- Cantaloupe
- Mango
- Peaches
- Asparagus
- Romaine lettuce
- Tomatoes
- Leafy greens
- Squash
- Whole grains
- Potatoes
- bananas
- Lentils
- Chili peppers
- Peas
- Apricots
- Tomatoes
- Papaya
- Red Bell Peppers
- Dandelions
- Liver
- Mackerel
- Pork
- Nuts
- Seeds
- Grapefruit
- Oysters
- Oily fish
- Cheeses
- Avocado

Vitamin B1

Vitamin B1 aka Thiamine is super important in the production of energy. It helps our bodies cells convert carbohydrates into energy. It is essential for the functioning of the heart, muscles, and nervous system. Not getting enough thiamine can leave one **fatigued and weak.**

*Most fruits and vegetables are not a significant source of thiamine so we get these gems from our **nuts, grains, proteins and beans.**

Foods highest in B1 are; pork, oysters, green peas, lima beans, salmon, tuna, pork, chia seeds, pumpkins seeds, squash seeds, pecans, cashews, pistachios, whole wheat, rye, corn, butternut squash, acorn squash, asparagus, black beans, edamame

Vitamin B2

Vitamin B2 aka Riboflavin functions as a coenzyme. Meaning that some of the properties created in our body need Riboflavin to help the do their jobs. What that means is they are helpful best friends with our bodies.

- They help produce red blood cells, which are incredibly important! They are responsible for carrying the oxygen our lungs absorb through breathing to every little part of our bodies.

- They help break down the calories we get from the protein, carbs and fats we eat. When our bodies break down these three macro-nutrients it creates usable energy for our body to use and boosts our **metabolism!**

- They also help metabolize the pharmaceutical drugs we take. With out Riboflavin. In fact only some drugs will only work when processed by riboflavin. It is also responsible for metabolizing drugs out of our systems to help prevent overdoses.

- They also help activate **antioxidants** to fight off oxidation.(I will get more into antioxidants later)

****So basically these are awesome little warriors that have so many different functions, that we can't take them lightly, **energy production, immune function and iron absorption.**

Foods highest in B2 are; leafy greens, broccoli, cauliflower, brussel sprouts, peppers, root vegetables, squash, mushrooms, whole grains, almonds, liver, wild rices, soybeans, poultry

Vitamin B3

Vitamin B3 aka Niacin: is also the body make various sex and stress-related hormones in the adrenal glands and other parts of the body. Niacin helps improve circulation, and it has been shown to suppress inflammation.

Symptoms of MILD niacin deficiencies are; *fatigue, depression, circulation problems, indigestion, vomiting, canker sores*
Symptoms of SERIOUS deficiency is Pellagra; *cracked scaly skin, diarrhea and dementia*

Natural Foods highest in B3; meat, liver, peanuts, mushrooms, cantaloupe, mango, peaches, asparagus romaine lettuce, tomatoes, mustard greens, squash, whole grains, potatoes, bananas, lentils, chili peppers, beans, yeast and molasses

Vitamin B5

Vitamin B5 aka Pantothenic Acid is essential to help the body use fats and protein. It is needed for healthy skin, hair, eyes, and liver. B5 is critical in creating red blood cells, as well as sex and stress-related hormones produced in the adrenal glands. It also helps synthesize cholesterol and helping the nervous system function properly.
This is a vitamin we need to replenish everyday, it is not stored. It is in all the other food groups as the rest of the Vitamin B's.

Good sources for B5 aka Pantothenic acid; avocado, grapefruit, guava, pomegranate, raspberries, watermelon, star-fruit, dates, mushrooms, cheese, oily fish, eggs, pork, veal, beef, chicken, turkey, sunflower seeds, sweet potatoes

Vitamin B6

Vitamin B6 helps to create antibodies for our **immune system.** It helps maintain **normal nerve function** and acts in the formation of red blood cells. It is also required for the chemical reactions of proteins. The higher the protein intake, the more need there is for vitamin B6. Too little B6 in the diet can cause dizziness, nausea, confusion, irritability and convulsions.

Foods highest in B6 are; Sunflower seeds, sesame seeds, flax seed, pumpkin, squash seeds, pistachios, hazelnuts, peanuts, macadamia nuts, walnuts, cashews, wild salmon, swordfish, halibut, tuna, turkey, chicken, lean beef, sirloin, rib-eye steak, pork, dried prunes, dried apricots, raisins, bananas, avocado, spinach.

Vitamin B9

Vitamin B9 aka Folic Acid along with the other B vitamins, helps the body to break down and convert the food that we eat into energy. It is needed to create and maintain cells. It helps make amino acids, red blood cells, DNA and RNA and is especially important during pregnancy. It helps prevent heart disease and stroke. A deficiency in Folic Acid constitutes to depression, rectal cancer and **BREAST CANCER.**

Foods high in B9 aka Folic Acid; asparagus, avocado, dark leafy greens, broccoli, citrus fruits, strawberries, raspberries, green beans, peas, navy beans, black beans, pinto beans, lentils, okra, brussel sprouts, flax seed, peanuts, sunflowers seeds, almonds,cauliflower, corn, beets, celery, carrots, squash.

Vitamin B12

Vitamin B12 aka cobalamin is a water-soluble vitamin that has a **key role in the normal functioning of the brain and nervous system via the synthesis of myelin,** and the formation of red blood cells. It is involved in the metabolism of every cell of the human body, especially affecting the creation of DNA, fatty acid and amino acid metabolism. **Getting B12 daily is crucial as we age, since deficiency is linked to cognitive decline and impaired nerve function.**

Fun Fact: *No fungi, plants, or animals are capable of producing vitamin B. We are pretty damn amazing.*

Food High in B12 are; shrimp, swiss cheese, sardines, mussels, milk, clams, beef, chicken, eggs, oysters, yeast, turkey, crab, salmon, trout, herring, octopus, custard, beef ribs, corned beef, scallops, mozzarella

Vitamin C

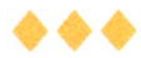

Vitamin C helps protect cells and keep them healthy. Vitamin C is also important because it helps protect the fat-soluble Vitamin A and Vitamin E as well as fatty acids from oxidation. (I go over oxidation in a later section) Vitamin C prevents and cures the disease scurvy, and can be beneficial in the treatment of iron deficiency anemia . It's also helps in the production of collagen, healthy connective tissues, supports structures of tissues and organs like , skin, blood vessels and bones. It is important in wound healing and it helps us absorb more iron from iron rich foods. It does an awesome job at helping stave of sickness and disease (ie..colds), and it an an amazing antioxidant. Vitamin C is a water-soluble vitamin and must be replenished everyday.

Foods rich in Vitamin C

- Cantaloupe
- Water cress
- Cabbages
- Collard greens
- Grapefruit
- Swiss chard
- Gooseberries
- Spinach
- Mango
- Blackberries
- Raspberries
- Potatoes
- Peas
- Tomatoes
- Turnips
- Cherries
- Apricots
- Rose hips
- Guava
- Yellow Bell Peppers
- Red Bell Peppers
- Parsley
- Kale
- Kiwi
- Broccoli
- Brussel sprouts
- Papaya,
- Strawberries
- Oranges
- Lemons & limes, clementines, pineapple,cauliflower

Vitamin D

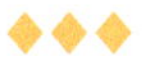

Vitamin D refers to a group of fat-soluble secosteroids responsible for increasing intestinal absorption of calcium, magnesium, and phosphate. In humans, the most important compounds in this group are vitamin D3 and vitamin D2. Only a few foods contain vitamin D. The major natural source of the vitamin is synthesis of cholecalciferol in the skin from cholesterol through a chemical reaction that is dependent on sun exposure. Our body must have vitamin D to absorb calcium and promote bone growth. Too little vitamin D results in soft bones in children (rickets) and fragile, misshapen bones in adults.

Vitamin D is needed to keep muscles, teeth and strong healthy bones. Although it has health benefits that are most commonly associated with bone health, it is also involved in supporting the immune and nervous systems, as well as brain function. It helps regulate the immune system and the neuromuscular system. It also plays major roles in the life cycle of human cells.

True Fact: *Vitamin D is so important that your body makes it by itself -- <u>but only after skin exposure to sufficient sunlight.</u>*

Vitamin E

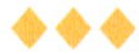

To change your life, you need to change your priorities
~unknown

Vitamin E is an antioxidant. This means it protects body tissue from damage caused by substances called free radicals, which can harm cells, tissues, and organs. They are believed to play a role in certain conditions related to aging, fatigue and headaches. The body also needs **vitamin E** to help keep the **immune system** strong against viruses and bacteria. Vitamin E boosts the immune system and helps the body fight germs. Vitamin E also keeps blood vessels open wide enough for blood to flow freely, and it helps the cells of the body work together to perform many important functions.

Foods rich in Vitamin E

- Almonds
- Nuts
- Seeds
- Vegetable oils
- Green leafy vegetables
- Spinach
- Avocados
- Squash
- Kiwi
- Tomato
- Sweet Potatoe
- Hazelnut
- Carrot Juice
- Broccoli
- Wheat germ oil
- Olive oil
- Shrimp
- Trout

Vitamin K

Vitamin K helps with blood coagulation so when we cut or puncture our skin we don't bleed out. It helps with cardiovascular health, the hardening of our arteries and helps to prevent osteoporosis. It is the "director" of calcium to places like our bones, making them stronger & helping to repair them and to our teeth to help prevent cavities. It also prevents calcium from going to the wrong areas, such as to your kidneys, where it could lead to kidney stones, or your blood vessels, where it could trigger heart disease.

It benefits sex by increasing testosterone and fertility in men, and decreasing the hormones in women who have with poly-cystic ovarian syndrome. It helps in creating insulin to stabilize our blood sugar, which helps prevent diabetes and metabolism problems like obesity. It works wonders suppressing genes that can promote cancers all while strengthening the genes that promote healthy genes. Enhancing your ability to utilize energy as you exercise improving overall performance.

Foods rich in Vitamin K

- Basil
- Swiss chard
- Lamb
- Water cress
- Turnips
- Collard greens
- Endive
- Brussel sprouts
- Broccoli
- Asparagus
- Leeks
- Okra
- Fennel
- Kale
- Spinach
- Mustard seed
- Parsley

Calcium

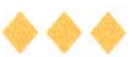

Small steps in the right direction are better than
big ones in the wrong direction.
~unknown

Calcium is a mineral that the body needs for building and maintaining bones and teeth, blood clotting, the transmission of nerve impulses, and the regulation of our heart's rhythm. Most of our calcium is stored in our bones which means that our bones are the first place we take our calcium from when our body is low in calcium. When that happens, it weakens our bones and makes us prone to osteoporosis, which mainly affects women.

In order for our body to transmit impulses signals to the nerves and brain, we need calcium and magnesium. They work together as partners. The conductor for these impulses is **calcium** which enters the cells through calcium channels operated by **magnesium**. Once calcium does its work, magnesium helps the body get rid of the calcium before it crystallizes. If not enough magnesium is present, then calcium builds up in the cells causing symptoms such as **hypertension**, **migraines** and **asthma**. The most important benefits of calcium and magnesium when we have adequate amounts of each are the are the following:

- Facilitation of **healthy blood pressure** and a steady heartbeat
- Prevention of **muscle cramps and pain**
- Support of the **nervous system** by ensuring fast transmission of messages all over the body

True Fact: *When our bodies are low in calcium it triggers our vitamin D to activate which then travels to our intestines (to encourage greater calcium absorption into the blood) and to our kidneys (to minimize calcium loss in the urine).*

Foods rich in Calcium

- Milk
- Yogurts
- Cheeses
- Tofu
- Black molasses
- Almond
- Kale
- Soybean
- Collard greens
- Spinach
- Chocolate (yep!)
- Rhubarb
- Chickpeas
- Garbanzo beans
- Egg Yolk
- Black-Eyed Peas

Iron

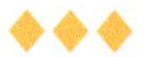

The Body Achieves what the Mind Believes
~unknown

Iron is extremely important in making red blood cells, which carry oxygen around the body. Without it, our cells would become starved for oxygen, our brain and muscles wouldn't function, and our **immune system would be impaired**, among other problems. It is also stored in the liver, spleen and bone marrow. A lack of **iron** can lead to anemia.

The twisted part about iron though, is that although it is absolutely necessary for a healthy body, there has been some grumbling about a tie to iron deposited in the brain and MS. This article abstract written by **James M. Stankiewicz, Mohit Neema, Antonia Ceccarelliby;** Department of Neurology, Brigham and Women's Hospital, Harvard Medical School, Partners Multiple Sclerosis Center, Brookline, MA, USA; ***Iron and multiple sclerosis*** is a great article to look up. Here is the abstract.

"Iron is essential for normal cellular functioning of the central nervous system. Abnormalities in iron metabolism may lead to neuronal death and abnormal iron deposition in the brain. Several studies have suggested a link between brain iron deposition in normal aging and chronic neurologic diseases,including multiple sclerosis (MS). In MS, it is still not clear whether iron deposition is an epiphe-nomenon or a mediator of disease processes. In this review, the role of iron in the pathophysiology of MS will be summarized. In addition, the importance of conventional and advanced magnetic reso-nance imaging techniques in the characterization of brain iron deposition in MS will be reviewed.Although there is currently not enough evidence to support clinical use of iron chelation in MS, an overview of studies of iron chelation or antioxidant therapies will be also provided."

Foods rich in Calcium

- Clams
- Oysters
- Soybeans
- Live
- Pumpkin seeds
- Beans
- Lentils, spinach

- Spinach
- Red Meat
- Poultry
- Seafood

Zinc

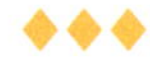

Zinc is found in cells throughout the body. **It is needed for the body's immune system to properly work.** It plays a role our cell division, cell growth, wound healing, and the breakdown of our carbohydrates. Zinc is also needed for the senses of smell and taste.

Zinc is an essential mineral that stimulates the activity of about 100 enzymes in the body. It also:

- supports your healthy immune system
- is necessary to synthesize DNA
- is essential for wound healing.
- supports the healthy growth and development of the body during adolescence, childhood and pregnancy.

Though the actual amount of zinc necessary to support the human body is small, its effects on the body are incredible.

Foods rich in Zinc

- Oysters
- Beans
- Dark Chocolate
- Cashews
- Whole wheat
- Pumpkin seed
- Sunflower seeds
- Shiitake mushrooms
- Beef
- Lentils
- Wild rice,
- Spinach
- Lamb
- Pecans
- Maple Syrup
- Crab
- Almonds
- Cocoa Beans
- Barley
- Peanuts
- Cheese
- Walnuts

Chromium

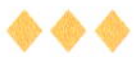

Chromium helps prevent cardiovascular disease which is awesome, but I am excited about its good effect on insulin which helps prevent type II diabetes. You see, our consumption of sugars and junk foods increases the amount of insulin your body must release into your blood stream, chromium helps by making us more sensitive to insulin and therefore helping to remove all that excess sugar, but this causes us to use up the chromium in our bodies, which is why it is very important to ingest a lot of chromium. (if you have seen Erin Brockovich, don't worry, this form is good for us)

Foods rich in Chromium

- Apples
- Sweet potatoes
- Corn
- Eggs
- Tomatoes
- Broccoli
- Herbs
- Whole grains
- Brown rice
- Mushrooms
- Green Beans
- Yeast
- Beef
- Chicken
- Fish
- Seafood
- Cheese
- Milk
- Dairy Products

Potassium

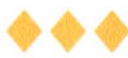

Potassium is an essential nutrient used to maintain our fluids and electrolyte balance. It controls the electrical activity of our hear,t our bodies also needs it to build proteins, break down and use carbohydrates, and to maintain the pH balance of our blood. It is very good for children because it helps support healthy growth. A deficiency in potassium causes fatigue, irritability, and high blood pressure.

Foods rich in Potassium

- Bananas
- Beef
- Fish
- Chicken,
- Cantaloupe
- Potatoes
- Tomatoes
- Lima beans
- White beans
- Acorn squash
- Spinach
- Low fat yogurt
- Salmon
- Apricots
- Mushrooms
- Seafood
- Avocado

Sodium

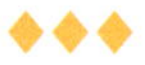

Eat Good. Feel Good.
~unknown

Sodium, we know it as a mineral the can our risk for high blood pressure, but our body needs sodium to stimulate nerve and muscle function, maintain the correct balance of fluid in the cells and support the absorption of other nutrients. Himalayan salt is my go too! It is also helps control blood sugar levels, it is a natural antihistamine, balances our bodies PH, helps with sleep, increases our metabolism, supports thyroid functions, and balancing our hormones!

Foods rich in Sodium

- Green Vegetables
- Leafy Vegetables
- Beet root
- Fruits
- Fish
- Meat
- Himalayan salt
- Whole meal flour
- Celery
- Bananas
- Water
- Milk
- Beans

Magnesium

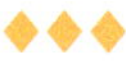

Don't start a short-term diet.
Start a long-term LIFESTYLE CHANGE.
~Danielle Vonn Brandt

Magnesium is an essential mineral required used for maintaining normal muscle and nerve function, keeping a healthy immune system, keeps our heart beating regularly, builds strong bones and boosts immunity. It works with calcium to transmit electrical nerve impulses. A deficiency in magnesium can lead to muscle spasms, cardiovascular disease, diabetes, high blood pressure, anxiety disorders, migraines, osteoporosis.

Foods rich in Magnesium

- Whole grains
- Avocados
- Yogurt
- Bananas
- Dried fruit
- Dark chocolate
- Green vegetables
- Peanut Butter
- Leafy greens
- Nuts
- Seeds
- Fish
- Beans

**Funny story about how our bodies are very good at communicating with us if we just knew how to listen. I used to hate peanut butter! I hated the sticky texture when I would eat it. I especially hated peanut butter and jelly sandwiches, I couldn't stand how it would stick to the roof of my mouth. I was basically a nightmare to pack a school lunch for as a child.

Ironically that year before I was diagnosed with MS (but I still knew something was wrong with me) I was craving peanut butter, very similar to a pregnancy craving but without the pregnancy. I would stand there in the kitchen eating peanut butter out of the container by the spoonful!
Well, it turns out that when I was hospitalized with my first MS attack they came in to tell me my blood work showed that I was anemic (I have always been anemic) and extremely low on magnesium. They recommended I take supplements and eat more broccoli and (get this) PEANUT BUTTER! I told them about the random cravings I had been having, apparently my body had been telling me I was low on magnesium. I have never had that issue in my past so I was surprised. To this day I regularly eat peanut butter, as I have grown a fondness.

So basically... Just remember that that we are not defined by our illness, we define ourselves. We do not fit into a neat and tidy box and only we can truly know our limits. We must search for them ourselves, as no one can tell us what they are. I am sharing this information with you because it has helped me immensely. I have seen and felt amazing changes in my body by even just cutting out free sugar. I hope that this will help you just as much as it has helped me.

Wake Up

◆◆◆

"Sometimes the people around you
won't understand your journey.
They don't need to, it's not for them."
~ Joubert Botha

OK, so we talked about looking at and changing our eating habits and why it is super important for our bodies to get the best nutrition we can give it and why we need to limit our free sugar intake and avoid artificial sweeteners and unhealthy fats. We are what we eat, so it is extremely important to know what we are putting into our bodies! Now I will explain what exercise has done for me after I stopped fearing it and stopped using my MS as a crutch.

Unfortunately I live in a very tiny rural village in Upstate New York known as Merrill. Now I am about 35 minutes—on a good day—from any type of urban amenities such as real grocery stores and stoplights, so it is a trek for me to go to the gym on a daily basis and I was never motivated to workout alone at home because I enjoy social interaction and I need accountability. I always had an excuse to fall back on whenever I got the whim to exercise, so all those fleeting moments came and went quickly.

My life partner William is one of the healthiest people that I know. He is in amazing shape and takes pride in fitness and exercise. He is my biggest supporter when it comes to my disease and he has always pushed me to break away from the way I looked at my MS. He pushes his limits everyday and encourages me to push past mine as well.

When I look back, I will admit that a lot of the "limitations" I had to break through were mostly fear and mental in regards to my physical abilities. No, I am not discounting physical symptoms from my MS but I will note that even some of my physical symptoms where not as severe as I had initially thought. For example, have you ever just sat down and start thinking about a weaker part of your body and you could actually feel the weakness— yet, when you are busy and not focusing on it, it really isn't as obvious in feeling that you thought? I find that when I am talking about my MS or I'm at the doctors office my symptoms seem to be very obvious to me, but in everyday life, when I am not thinking about my MS or letting it consume my days I hardly notice it. On the outside people have no idea I have MS unless I tell them. Once I was able to recognize that, I was able to excel and flourish.

It just happened one day, I woke up exhausted with my current life, I literally woke up and it was like something had flipped a switch in my brain. I was done! A couple friends of mine from back home—Port Orchard, WA—had gotten really involved in fitness and diet lifestyle changes and it got me thinking and motivated me to try something new in my life. I was sick of being a "victim" and I hated who I was letting my MS make me become, so I got more information on how to take that first step that would change my life and help me take back the control I thought I had lost since MS showed up.

Don't Follow the
Yellow Brick Road

◆◆◆

Don't let your MS tell you which
way to go...Take your own path.
~Danielle Vonn Brandt

So, I took a right at the fork in the road on the journey of my life. I took the path less traveled and just kept marching forward. I was extremely overwhelmed and a little freaked out but what could I lose? Nothing! I needed to do this, I needed a change and wanted to have control in my life again. I was sick of "surviving" everyday.

For me, this new path lead me to Beach Body and fell in love with the way it made me feel, with the way that exercising made me feel and I loved the accountability groups! This is the journey that lead me to look more into to my eating habits and the what and why of what my body needed.

Please note that I am not trying to sell you on Beach Body, I promise!

It is a great program for me but it may not be for you. Their easy access to all the types of programs at anytime and anywhere is what made my life easier—I don't have a gym next door to me— and the on-line accountability and challenge groups helped fill my need for accountability, I had found something that worked for me. Any program that promotes fitness and exercise will work. Join a gym near you, find a local Cross Fit or YMCA, start dancing, swimming, running, or even just walking everyday. Just get moving, that is all you need to do.

Finally, I was able to stay focused and be held accountable. I could workout at home or at the park I took my youngest daughter to or even at work when I had time available. I had an accountability group I connected with and they helped keep me pushing through the hard days. I had access to tons of programs for every level and ability—which I found helped fit better into my person fitness level and allowed me to grow and change it up. I felt myself getting stronger, I wasn't as tired anymore and I was a noticeably happier person. I had not felt this good in such a long time. The change I felt in me was and is amazing. I got stronger everyday and pushed myself. I found that the more I pushed my limits, the more mental barriers I broke through. Like I said earlier, most of the limitations we have are ones we create in our minds. The freedom I felt was blissful—I could feel the control coming back, finding its way out of the chaos MS had created 10 years earlier.

The Brains Behind the Matter!

◆◆◆

The FEARS we don't face,become our
LIMITS and WEAKNESSES.
Be BRAVE
~Danielle Vonn Brandt

Lets stop and take at look at what makes exercise so important and what effects it has on our brains. Exercise has been stated to help treat depression, improve memory loss, and benefits diseases such as Alzheimer's, Dementia and Multiple Sclerosis. Exercise helps trigger the release of certain neurotransmitters in our brains that helps reduce mental and physical pain and—this is pretty amazing—it is one of the few ways scientists have found that adults can generate new neurons. All types of cardio exercises provide benefits– because when we exercise it starts a type of domino effect on the brain through several mechanisms including neurogenesis, stabilizing depression, releasing endorphins which causes us to feel happier and helping to improve cognitive functioning. What I find to be the most exciting change that exercise causes is neurogenesis or the birth of new neurons. New undamaged neurons, with all their new possibilities. Can they really integrate and replace the damaged and dead cells in our brains? Apparently sciences is showing that they do start to integrate into our brains and become a part of the whole system.

But how? Lets take a peak at an article I came across in my research written by Dr. Douglas Fields, called **How Exercise Can Stimulate the Birth of New Neurons**;

It took decades of research to persuade scientists to give up their long-held belief that new neurons could not be formed in the brains of adults, but there is no longer any doubt about it. It is now well-established that strenuous physical exercise stimulates the birth of new neurons in part of the brain that is critical for memory, the hippocampus. The molecular and cellular details explaining how exercise stimulates the birth of new brain cells have been worked out now in great detail. Immature non-neuronal cells in the adult brain (glia) respond to protein growth factors that are generated in the body during robust physical activity. These growth factors stimulate the mother cells to spawn new neurons in the hippocampus. Amazingly, these nubile neurons then migrate through brain tissue to find their proper place in the neural circuitry. Even more remarkable, new research proves that the new neurons are then able to wire themselves into the existing network of connections to boost performance in memory, just like adding RAM chips does for a laptop....Why should pumping muscles build more brain cells? ...explain the odd connection between burning calories and birthing neurons....Building brains by exercise has been shown to provide animals with an increased cognitive reserve, meaning that after brain injury or disease that kills or damages healthy neurons, animals that have been forced to do reps on the exercise wheel before a brain injury, do far better in recovering. The animals forced to work out also have much slower cognitive decline in aging compared to sedentary cage-mates, because the loss of brain cells is a normal process of aging. Surprisingly, the same drugs used to treat chronic depression have been found to stimulate the birth of new neurons in the hippo campus. This ancient biological connection between muscle and brain can account for how pumping iron could benefit our mental health as well as our cognitive health; not to mention the side effect of shaping legs and flattening bellies.

Now that is crazy!! I was extremely shocked when I read that, but honestly our bodies are capable of so much that we don't even realize. With the right combination of choices, our bodies will behave differently and adapt to those changes. Putting the right nutrients into our bodies and giving our bodies the right amount exercise has such beneficial reactions as, weight loss, more energy, strength, self healing, reducing diseases such as diabetes, heart disease, dementia, Alzheimer's and MS.

Now I am 5'9, slender and I have always considered myself to be on the healthy side! I had always thought of myself as a pretty good eater but I did slack on exercising since my MS diagnoses in 2008. I am 33 years old and working in the medical field I had noticed that my heart rate was a little wonky. My resting heart rate even in my late 20's was a slightly tachycardic, meaning, that my resting heart rate was faster that normal, but after just 2 months of getting a little exercise everyday, my resting heart rate is now within the normal defined limits of 60-90 bpm.

I have now come to realize that there is so much that I did not know or understand about my body or nutrition at all. Well, thanks to technology and the ability to understand my body better, I have a much better sense of things. I have been more adamant about wanting to know the whys and what-ifs. I wanted to step outside of my neat little box I had been stuffed into and try to make sense of what I could do to make myself stronger and healthier. I wanted to give myself a better chance at being happy and healthy again. So lets go over the what and why in the physical fitness area.

Fitness=Happiness

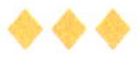

You don't have to be fast,
you just have to go.
~unknown

So how do all of these benefits of exercising explain the blissful and happier state I felt after even just a solid 15 minute workout? And if it has such a huge impact on my brain, what does it do to the other aspects of my body? Well, when we first start working out it it will feel awkward and a bit hard. I mean hard as in your heart rate will increase and you will begin to breathe deeper, heavy and faster. **This is normal.** Your body is adjusting to all the activity you are doing that it is not used to. When your breathing increases and your heart rate goes up, that is your bodies way of getting more oxygen to your muscles. When we breathe air into our lungs, they absorb the oxygen and transfers it over to our heart to pump through our body which in return lowers our heart rate.

But, we are not only working out our muscles when we are exercising, in the process we are making our hearts stronger and bigger. This means that our heart rate lowers because it can get more done with less effort. And not only does it strengthen our hearts but it causes our blood vessels to become more elastic, which helps lower our blood pressure! Exercising also delivers more oxygen to our brains which helps release the hormones that help with cell growth.

In regards to helping our brains create new neurons, any cardiovascular exercises, some examples are running, walking at a brisk pace, interval training such as Cross-fit, (my favorites) ShaunT or Core DE Force and yoga are the single most effective ways of boosting neurogenesis. They also come with a vast array of health benefits for mind and body, and are also important stress relievers. The endorphins that our bodies are producing during a workout act as strong warriors against cortisol, which is our stress hormone—we all know what stress does to us— and it has been found to increase levels of the two growth factors that support neurogenesis, BDNF (brain derived neurotrophic factor) and GDNF (glial cell line-derived trophic factor). Please don't ask me to get more in depth. I am not a scientist.

Just Do It

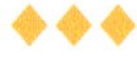

Everybody can spare 15-30 minutes a day to devote to being active! It can even be fun. I know the start can be overwhelming, but you will adjust! You will see that you become a little bit better then you were the day before. It is addicting. My absolute favorite program and the one that I started with was 21 Day Fix. I felt capable and that felt amazing in itself!. It made me stronger and happier, it reduced my fatigue and I was actually excited to do week two. Eventually I finished 21 Day Fix and started doing Core DE Force. That is a cardio program that uses MMA and boxing style moves— so I felt like a total bad-ass, I liked it so much I became an instructor. Ultimately, I lost about 25-30 lbs and felt amazing and confident and strong—weight loss was not the only goal but it is an amazing benefit. I had taken control of what I could control. I have learned to nurture my body with healthy foods and to strengthen my body with exercise. I started to notice that mentally I looked at the world differently, I didn't feel weak and scared of all the tomorrows anymore.

Let your body move! It needs to move and it wants to move. We are not meant for just sitting. We are pretty amazing creatures and are capable of doing more that any other creature on earth. We can't take our abilities to move and feel for granted, because we are going to miss them incredibly if we lose them. No matter your physical ability there is always something you can do to strengthen your body.

What Happens

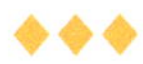

Don't give up because of one bad chapter in your life.
Keep going...your story doesn't end here.
~unknown

Well, if we look back to how physically active we are in this day in age and compare ourselves to even just 75 years ago, then we are lazy and boring. Even washing laundry was a very physical task. Our society today is all about easy and convenient but it is hurting us physically. Our bodies are meant to move and stay active, but today the more we don't have to move the more enjoyable we perceive our lives to be. The more sedentary we are the more unhealthy we become and the more we are at risk of diseases —that have basically become a common ailment in our country—such as diabetes, cardiovascular problems, obesity—which leads to being even more sedentary because of the difficulty and pain of the moving around—which leads to surgery on joints and the cycle continues. All of the conveniences we have available to us are awesome if we use some of that time to be active in other ways, go for a hike or a walk,. join a group of friends and do something fun and active together.

We have the ability and the capacity to understand our bodies in a way that we never have had before. So not only do we now understand that certain life style choices can lead us to early death or disability, but we are more enlightened as to why we should be exercising more and understanding what our bodies require to stay healthy for our lifetime. Lets look at it this way, our bodies are the vehicle or machine to our mind/brain and we need to maintain it or our machine will break-down and may not be repairable. How can we look the other way about our lives and our health when the knowledge is right there for us to use. We have access to all the tools we need to start maintaining our health and bettering our bodies, this includes our daily eating habits, exercising our bodies and strengthening our minds.

Feeling Sexy

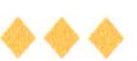

Remember that the reason you are
doing this is to make your life better.
~unknown

Sex is beneficial for brain function while elevating levels of feel good neurotransmitters and promoting neurogenesis. I know that sexual appetite can decrease with MS but just do it! You will always feel glorious after, I promise! It also help us to sleep better. Your body releases oxytocin, also called the "love" hormone, and endorphins during an orgasm. The combination of these hormones can act as a sleep inducer. Better sleep patterns lead to a stronger immune system, longer lifespan and feeling well rested with more energy throughout the day.

Another study shows that sexual activity can provide full or partial relief from migraines and cluster headaches, whether they are associated with our MS or not. I know from personal experience that if I was starting to feel a migraine coming on and I was able to have sex and orgasm that it wouldn't hit me. About 70 percent of people reported moderate to complete relief during a migraine. 91 percent of people reported moderate to complete relief in cluster headaches. So whether you are able to have sex or give yourself an orgasm, that is a huge relief.

Catch some ZZZ's

◆◆◆

Get up every morning and remind
yourself that you can do this!
~Danielle Vonn Brandt

While we MS Warriors know that we can always use plenty of sleep and usually take it when we can get it, it has been shown that sleep deprivation reduces neurogenesis. In regards to getting the sleep we need when our bodies demand it, research suggests that sleep is key to our brain being able to detox itself. I never knew that our brains did that and I am almost wondering what the connection is to our extreme fatigue symptoms with MS and our brain toxins. Are our brains creating more toxins because of all the extra work it has to do? Does the build up of toxins contribute to the fatigue we fight on a regular basis?

Dr. Maiken Nedergaard, co-director of URMC's Center for Translational Neuromedicine, says:

".. study shows that the brain has different functional states when asleep and when awake. In fact, the restorative nature of sleep appears to be the result of the active clearance of the by-products of neural activity that accumulate during wakefulness....The brain only has limited energy at its disposal and it appears that it must [choose] between two different functional states - awake and aware or asleep and cleaning up. You can think of it like having a house party. You can either entertain the guests or clean up the house, but you can't really do both at the same time."

Basically, there is an importance in regards to sleeping and the length of time our bodies need to sleep. What happens to our brains when our "machines" are sleeping, it is very much still at work,but, it is enjoying "quiet time" while it cleans the house. (You understand quiet time if you are a parent or deal with children on a regular basis. I, in fact, very much value my personal quiet time!)

During our sleep cycle, the part of our brain called the glymphatic system and it's glial cells clears away toxins and waste products that could be responsible for brain diseases, like Alzheimer's and other neurological disorders. Apparently our glymphatic system is actually 10 times more active during sleep, the brain even undergoes physical changes that allows the system to work faster. Brain cells shrink by 60%, increasing the space between them so the toxins can be flushed away more effectively.

The "F" Word
FATIGUE

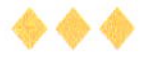

Why is fatigue such an issue with MS patients? While I know from personal experience that on a "bad fatigue day" it can be extremely difficult to try and function normally for even small amounts of time, it makes easy mundane tasks much more challenging. Fatigue is considered by many of us to be the worst part of our MS and unfortunately, it affects most of us. The worst part about our fatigue is that it does not generally improve with rest or sleep. And that feeling of being physically and mentally weak and walking around like we are in a "brain fog." doesn't help at all.

Scientists don't know for sure if there is an exact link between our nerve damage and fatigue, but some studies have suggested that certain parts of the brain are linked to fatigue. There have not been any single areas of the brain identified yet and I am not sure if I really buy into that concept. But another suggestion that makes a little more sense is that the fatigue we feel might be caused by the way that our brains adapt to the impact of the MS itself.

MRI scans of people who have fatigue show that they use larger areas of the brain to carry out activities than people who don't have fatigue and it may be due to the damage in several areas of the brain or spinal cord from our attacks. Perhaps the brain is finding new routes for messages when the usual nerve paths have been damaged and finding new routes might mean it takes more energy to carry out an action—which in return may cause the fatigue.

It is known that fatigue is commonly worsened when our body temperatures rise—like on a hot day, have a fever, or take a hot bath —but don't worry too much if this happens. When heat worsens our fatigue, it's not a sign of a new relapse and is reversible when the heat source is removed. Just be prepared for hot weather and stay hydrated.

What you Feed Yourself

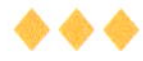

This refers to the beginning of the book, but lets reiterate, that our diet plays an important role in brain health and neurogenesis. Excessive Free sugar(refined sugars) has a negative effect on our brain, and refined and processed foods should be avoided as well. The brain is made of significant amounts of fats and water, which is why it is so important to consume enough of each. The right fats are essential to healthy brain function, these require a certain amount of plant and animal fats. Studies have found that omega 3 fatty acids are important in regards to neurogenesis and these healthy fatty acids are a major structural component of the brain and many other parts of the body.

Other things such as consuming antioxidants like blueberries, dark chocolate, tea, red wine and cannabinoids are also beneficial to brain health and supportive of neurogenesis. Some foods have more direct effects on the process, such as the spice turmeric. Curcumin is the main active compound in the spice, and has been found to increase BDNF (that big scientific word) levels while acting as an antidepressant with an effectiveness of antidepressant drugs but without their side effects.

A variety of other lifestyle factors influence neurogenesis. Exposure to sunlight is well known for its role in increasing vitamin D, but it also increases serotonin levels and GDNF(that other big scientific word) in the brain. Exposure to sunlight is healthy, if exposure times are limited to times of day when it is safest to do so, when exposure to UV rays is reduced. Even just a brief exposure of around ten minutes to the face can have a positive effect on the brain.

Cannabis

◆◆◆

Cannabis—more commonly known as marijuana, has become very relevant in regards to alleviating some of the medical problems associated with MS. Cannabis is a naturally occurring drug made from parts of the cannabis plant and it has been used throughout history for medicinal purposes. Cannabis contains many different compounds which are known as cannabinoids but the two most well known cannabinoids that are studied for their potential medicinal effects are tetrahydrocannabinol (THC) and cannabidiol (CBD).

The most important thing to grasp is that THC will get you high and CBD will not. THC has psychoactive properties that affect your brain and give you that "high" while CBD is the medicinal aspect. So long story short, you can still take cannabis without the severe side effects of the high, although THC does have medicinal qualities as well. It has been shown that CBD may have a positive effect on neurogenesis, and studies show that it helps reduce anxiety and has anti-depressant behaviors associated with its use. CBD and THC are also well-known to relieve pain, reduce muscle spasms and help with migraines.

They have neuro-protective properties and they combat oxidative stress and protects our cells, tissues, and DNA from damage. The antioxidant, anti-inflammatory, and neuro-genetic qualities in this plant make it one powerful brain-boosting medicine. It's quite miraculous, really and becoming more and more available recognized for treatments all over the world.

Antioxidants vs. Oxidative Stress

While looking into cannabis and all the affects is can have, I started seeing *oxidative stress* a lot. I had to school myself in that process and what it is and what it does to our bodies. The process of *oxidation* happens as our bodies process the oxygen that we breathe and our cells produce energy from it. This process also produces free radicals (a molecule that isn't complete) – which interact with the molecules within our cells resulting in damage or stress to nearby cells and

DNA (our genes).

Free radicals are normal and necessary in our bodies in small amounts. Although they cause some damage, they also stimulate repair. It is only when there are more free radicals produced that they hinder the repair processes that it becomes an issue. That is what we call **oxidative stress.** Oxidation happens under a number of circumstances including: when our cells use glucose to make energy, *when the immune system is fighting off bacteria and creating inflammation* and when our bodies detoxify pollutants, pesticides, and cigarette smoke.

Oxidative stress causes **fatigue, memory loss and/or brain fog,** muscle and/or joint pain, wrinkles and gray hair, decreased eye sight, **headaches and sensitivity to noise and susceptibility to infections.** Oxidations causes our bodies to age much more quickly. If you compare long-term nicotine smokers to non-smokers you will see a big difference in their aging stages. While food is a huge source for our antioxidants we need to fight this process, CBD has been found to be as powerful, if not more so. Cannabis is a powerful antioxidant.

Anti-Inflammatory

While inflammation is an essential response by the body's immune system to injury, bacteria and viruses, at times the inflammatory response is called upon when it is not needed. When called upon appropriately, the inflammatory response effectively removes the infectious or damaging stimuli so that the body can initiate the healing process. However, when not officially needed, in the case of autoimmune diseases, the immune system reacts as if tissues are infected or abnormal when in actuality they are normal. As a result, the body causes damage to its own tissues. Acute inflammation that comes and goes as necessary to deal with injuries and diseases represents a well-balanced and effective immune system. With chronic inflammation, however, the immune system has essentially gone rogue and it won't shut off the inflammatory response.

What I find interesting are the effects that cannabis has shown in regards to its anti-inflammatory affects on MS. Cannabis has been known to reduce inflammation, and has been used as an anti-inflammatory for thousands of years all over the world. Recently, the ability of cannabis to reduce MS-related inflammation has been studied. A drug that was largely frowned upon in the past has stepped up its game in the medical field and doctors and scientists are starting to take it seriously.

It has been concluded that the presence of CBD and THC in our bodies prevents our immune cells from triggering the production of inflammatory molecules— which limits the molecules from reaching the brain and spinal cord and causing damage. High CBD containing strains are preferable in regards to brain health, and to get the most out of cannabis. A good way to consume CBD without any THC is to consume the CBD Oil orally or use a vaporizer. These are also the most effective and healthy ways to take it medicinally.

Finding our Inner Peace

◆ ◆ ◆

Inner peace begins the moment you
choose not to allow another person
or event to control your emotions.
~Pema Chodron

Through all the chaos and uncertainty in our daily lives because of MS, with all the erratic and unpredictable symptoms and side effects, we need to find a goodness in everyday. We need to control our minds and our outlook on our lives. We need to be able to accept ourselves and our bodies, we need to find peace. Peace is not the absence of a conflict, peace is the acceptance of conflict.

I learned from my decade of dealing with my MS that I needed to compartmentalize my stresses, I needed to learn how to better deal with them. I needed to first find peace with myself and my disease so that I could start taking control of my stress. I know from experience that stress exacerbate the symptoms of my MS because I was caught in a never ending motion of stress and fear, only to make matters that much worse, the cycle just wouldn't stop. I felt as though I was stuck in a never ending spiral and I never got a break. Finally I was tired of feeling weak and fragile.

Once I started to see the pattern, once I started looking at all of this chaos from a different perspective, I realized that I was the only one who could control my chaos and stress. I was the only one who could choose to control my stressful situations in a different way. Once I was able to accept myself and my body, I learned how to compartmentalize my stresses. I started learning how to better deal with things.

Lets face it...life is fond of throwing curve balls at us when we least expect them. Work, marriage, children, education, medical issues, friendships, holidays, even something as trivial as driving down the road or the weather. We need to focus on how to better handle our stressers. Little things that we can do to make the big things seem small and the little things seem like nothing.

I how frustrating and difficult it can be, but stressing out about things we cannot control only makes everything worse. I have learned and am still learning how to take things with a grain of salt. Don't fight the punches, but roll with them. Life is life for everybody and everybody has stresses, our exception is that our stresses actually make us more sick.

Find something that centers you. Whether it is meditation, prayer, exercise, writing or even finding things to be grateful for each day, find something that grounds you. Find something that works for you. Get out of your comfort zone, because if stress controls your life right now, then your current comfort zone is not working for you. Try new things because out of all the things we can't control in our lives, we can control how we live our lives. How we react to our lives and MS. Finding whatever works to calm your mind will eventually help to control your health.

Positive Thinking

◆◆◆

Though we rarely get to choose our challenges, and the outcomes are often out of our control, the one area where we do have complete power is attitude. We have two choices, let each challenge rule us, or rise up and make the most of the situation. Stop and smell the roses, take a deep breath, having a positive attitude doesn't mean ignoring your reality or forcing yourself to pretend it is not there. It is acceptance.

Choose to look at the bigger picture. Is it worth the time and stress you are choosing to expend over it. We need to accept that life will always happen, it is how we respond that makes the difference. Remember how I said that "we are what we eat"? Well, how we deal with life and the effects we let it have over us is how we are going to continually feel on a regular basis.

The best way to counteract our negative reaction is through self-awareness. Learn to recognize when you slip into a depressive state and consciously stop yourself. When you start to recognize the reaction that you want to change, you will them have the power to control your emotions and change that reaction. Learning how to handle your stresses will not happen overnight, it is something that you will need to constantly work on.

Try writing in a journal everyday for a month, write about your day, along with your feelings and emotions. After your month is up, go back and read through your journal. When you read back through the month do you see a pattern? Do you notice a baseline reaction to stress? Is it just all the negative aspects of your day, or are there positive and good things noted in your journal? What do you seem to be focused on the most?

Now try writing in your journal for another month, but this time try to focus on gratitude, laughter, friendship, kindness, resilience, self-love and self-respect. What are you happy about? Did you ever find yourself losing control and letting stress take over your day or did you recognize it and choose to take a different path? Compare the two different months. What do you see? Is there a change in how you feel and how you are handling things? Do you feel better?

Having a positive outlook doesn't mean you're free from bad circumstances or that you are pretending that life is always great. What a positive attitude means is that you know how to deal with what life throws your way. That you choose to make the best of bad situation.

Life with a chronic illness isn't easy, but a positive attitude can help us along in our journeys and help lift us up over some of our daily struggles. Celebrate life, it can help you continue to see the positive and all of the great things you're doing in your life, in spite of the challenges and setbacks we may face tomorrow.

You are stronger then you believe. I know it. You just need to start believing it. Start looking up and stop looking down. We are capable of amazing things. What makes us more amazing is the fact that we have to overcome more than most. Let that be a positive thing to look at. Our challenges help us to grow. They make us stronger. Start being your own HERO. Only you can change your life.

⇛⟶ I decide to become the healthiest and strongest and the best that I can be!

⇛⟶ I took to heart that old saying "You are what you eat", and I eat as healthy as I can!

⇛⟶ I exercise everyday at a level my body will allow!

⇛⟶ Everyday I seek out personal development, because your body will only go as far as your mind will let it!

THE THING ABOUT BEING

BRAVE

IS IT DOESN'T COME WITH THE ABSENCE OF FEAR AND HURT. BRAVERY IS THE ABILITY TO LOOK FEAR AND HURT IN THE FACE AND SAY MOVE ASIDE, YOU ARE IN THE WAY.

~ Melissa Tumino